The Loneliest Whale
in the World

Also by Tom C. Hunley

Poetry Books

What Feels Like Love: New and Selected Poems
Here Lies
The State That Springfield Is In
Plunk
Octopus
The Tongue
Still, There's a Glimmer

Poetry Chapbooks

Abridged: Erasure Poems
Adjusting to the Lights
Scotch Tape World
Annoyed Grunt
Tom C. Hunley Greatest Hits
My Life as a Minor Character
Newspring
Losing My Luggage

Craft Books

The Poetry Gymnasium
Teaching Poetry Writing: A Five-Canon Approach

Nonfiction

Creative Writing Pedagogies for the Twenty-First Century
(co-edited with Dr. Alexandria Peary)

Short Film

You're Not Alone

The Loneliest Whale
in the World

Tom C. Hunley

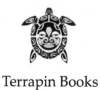

Terrapin Books

Terrapin Books
4 Midvale Avenue
West Caldwell, NJ 07006

www.terrapinbooks.com

ISBN: 978-1-947896-72-7
Library of Congress Control Number: 2023951585

First Edition

Cover art: Michael Kroetch
At the School for Special Children
Mixed media, 22" x 21"

Cover design: Diane Lockward

for Ralaina, Elizabeth, Evan, Owen, and Blake

Contents

I. Love as the World Ends

Commencement Address 7
People Yawn When Other People Yawn 8
Dear God, Show Me How to Walk in Wonder 10
Remember Those Girls, Lord 12
I never pushed my daughter 14
Love as the World Ends 17
Rock, Paper, Scissors Invent Calling Shotgun 20
Her Heart Was a Legend 21
Rock, Paper, Scissors Go to Therapy 23
Grace 24
Dirty Looks 25
Skinny Dipping 27
In My Man Cave 29
Only Son 31
Will Be Done 33

II. Between Worlds

The Last Time I Took My Son to the Movies 39
Adopting a Teenager Via State Foster Care 42
My Chili Recipe: An *Ars Poetica* 43
I See Your Lips Move, Lord 46
Two-Foot Tall Poem 48
What Will Survive 50
Rock, Paper, Scissors Reminisce 52
Stars in My Beard 53
Love Me Gentlefirm the Way Firemen Love
   a Treed Cat 54
My Sadness Swallows Up My Dreams 56
Fifty 57
At the Intersection of Yawn and Yawp 58
Between Worlds 59

Ankylosing Spondylitis   60
If This Next Apocalypse Gets Canceled
  or Postponed   62

III. A World Inside This World
A World Inside This World   67
If You've Met One Autistic Person,
  You've Met One Autistic Person   69
An Urn Among Music Boxes   70
Don't Try   74
To Make Light of the Dark   76
Body Breaking   77
The Man I Hoped to Be   78
Upon First Reading *Jesus' Son*
  by Denis Johnson   79
Rock, Paper, Scissors Want to be Called . . .   81
It's Not So Hard to Write a Sonnet, Man   82
I Regret Caring More About What People
  Think Than About People   83
Downloadable Caffeine   85
"and pain will be the thing that saves us."   87
Rock, Paper, Scissors Celebrate
  the End of the War   88
Questions for Further Study   89

Acknowledgments   93
About the Author   97

"O world, I cannot hold thee close enough!"
—Edna St. Vincent Millay, "God's World"

". . .We must get back to the real thing.
The blood and meat of the world."
—Ruth Stone, *Who Is the Widow's Muse* (#LII)

I. Love as the World Ends

Commencement Address

Now walk into a bar full
of nuns, cockroaches, and dragons.
Realize this is no joke.
Realize it's another classroom, not a bar.
Order a round for the house anyhow.
Learn from everyone.
Change habits.
Outlive the next war.
Breathe fire.
Don't take advice from anyone, poets especially,
but stay humble and open-minded.
If invited to give a commencement address,
keep it short
and don't make it about yourself.
Let joy inflict you.
Choose wanderlust.
Do cartwheels or fly in circles.
Waltz like a shy sunbeam
crawling across a wall
in search of a window to climb through.

People Yawn When Other People Yawn

but blush or look away
when other people cry.
All the heavy metal potheads
from high school became bankers
or lawyers or, in some cases,
well-heeled preachers.
Meanwhile, David Lee Roth,
formerly of Van Halen,
could show up at your door
to set up your DISH TV satellite
and you wouldn't even recognize him,
now would you? Or you'd recognize him,
but you'd yawn and he'd yawn
to hide the fact that he's crying inside.
Might as well jump
like a fish that shocks the air
and is shocked by it
before diving back
to its underwater world skimmed by sunlight.

Me, I've seen barbed wire rusting
in brittle morning light.
I've felt a horse's damp lips
graze my hand, heard its snort,
like wind flapping a flag.
Honest, I've heard a stadium exhale
as a ball landed in a glove, and I've spent

the car ride home trying to find
a way to describe that sound.
I've heard people laugh
when other people laugh
but it would be a lie to say,
I've never heard anyone laugh
as someone else cried. I need you
to know that the sky's
tilting from the heaviness
of all these southbound birds
but will right itself before you
have a chance to fact check me.

Dear God, Show Me
How to Walk in Wonder

Dear God, when I watched my firstborn
      being born, I thought, at first,
   he looked like a carp, hooked and gasping,
        and I was struck dumb, as silent as You.

My son couldn't speak for years,
      and when the doctor said *Autism*
  I couldn't speak, and forgive me,
      I turned my head from him.
I know You'll understand. Forgive me
      for reminding You how You turned Your head
        while Your son hung there.

Sometimes, God, I stumble like a foal,
      a fool, a fawn, a phony. I fail, I fall,
  I, who taught, by tall example,
      my children to walk.

Sometimes a wolf steps out of woods
      and I need new words
  to ward him off
    because the words I have
      have dried up in my throat.

Dear God, show me how to walk in wonder
      toward You and knock me over

when I walk away from You
but let me let my children
walk away from me.

Just remember the names I gave them:
She Who Fills My Head And Heart
With An Unshakeable Ache;
He Who Beats Drums And Beats Me At Ping Pong;
He Who Slaps The Bass And Cracks The Jokes;
and He Who Ventures Far Into The Cold

To A World Inside Himself
That No One Else Can Ever Enter.
Not even I can go there,
but I believe You can go there.
Dear God, please go there.

Remember Those Girls, Lord

Remember all those profiles of teen girls
in foster care, how we grieved
that we could only bring one home?
Remember those girls, Lord,
how the social workers advised:
this one bit her foster siblings
and is on lockdown; this one lit
a firecracker under a sleeping cat
and will soon age out of the system;
this one has falsely accused men and boys
in three foster homes and will ruin
your reputation; and this one (the one who
joined our family, thank you Lord)
ate shoplifted groceries with her
siblings as their birth mother
nodded off under the spell of heroin
and both men in her home
were unregistered sex offenders.

When some dirtboy sent dick pics
to her secret social media page,
how I raged, angry at him, afraid
for her. Lord, only You know
how many men and boys have shown her
their ugly sides. Composing myself,
I told her never to send pictures of her
body, but if she did, never to include her
face, because porn is a thing

and revenge porn is also a thing.
Thank You for keeping her off drugs—
but help me to see her
as myself at her age,
trembling in the county detox ward,
waiting for a room to open up
in a rehab center, and help me
be like the junkie I met there,
who said, *Hey, I only have one cigarette,
it's really all I have, but why don't you take it?*

I never pushed my daughter

in a stroller through the park
lost in a trance as the trees
seemed to listen as she

tried out sounds in hopes
of inventing words
for the warm feeling of

a full belly and a pink blanket
as a song rocked her to sleep.
Instead I read an online profile

that said she loved pets and
purple and singing and acting
and had hurts that I would have

to enter, scars like ravenous
mouths I couldn't escape
if I got close to her like

entering a mansion with
ghosts in it who don't
mind being dead but want

me to feel what they felt.
I never held her on my shoulders
up to the monkey bars

giggling, faux afraid of falling.
No, I got her after fire
got her, burned the world

she knew. I could see it
in her eyes. I felt like paper,
like if I touched her it would

torch me, but I told her
this would go away and come back
like traces of lightning bugs

growing fainter and more distant.
I watched *Instant Family* with her
over and over but only after

she had lived through scenes
she wasn't old enough
to see in movies.

I never tossed her
into the air, laughing,
sure I'd catch her

and if we played tag
a rolling boulder was *it*
and it wanted to flatten us

and if we played
hide-and-go-seek
we each hid in the darkness

surrounding us, neither
of us sure we'd
ever go free.

Love as the World Ends

'A': An honors student crams all night in case the test's not
     canceled.

Bison stampeding are rendered invisible by frost on windshields.

Children unborn, names already chosen, painted on cribs,
     blue and pink, smell of paint drying.

Dollars fall from the sky instead of rockets in our last dreams.

Everything done gets undone.

F: this.

Going, going, gonged.

Hungry for forgiveness, for another shot, for a last look from
     the bridge at the sparkling sun
          skimming the scalloped waves.

Ill: Kids say "sick" but mean something else. Al Gore said
     the world has a fever.

Just us: sacks of skin that want to touch and be touched,
     that want and wont and need and knead,
          sources of injustice, gathering places
               for goosebumps

Keep playing guitar. What song will you pick? You can't
keep anything. But if you could? What would you keep?

Like the simile, we're going the way of the Liaoceratops.

Making love might make us forget that we're about to explode,
might be the last come-on.

Anyway, this feels like the ultimate ultimatum.

Optimists, even the end of the world isn't the end
of the world to you.

Psalms are prayers that pop.

Cue the doomsday prophets, gleeful
about finally being right.

Re-reading Rimbaud in a ragged voice
sets the right mood for the day on fire.

Smoking: No reason not to start now.

There may not be there, depending on where we're going.

Underwear: Wear a clean pair.

Valery called perfume the refuse of flowers. Now you know that.

We were totally lied to by that REM song.

Exes: At least you won't bump into them in clubs any more.

Yesterday we said *yes* and *yes* and yet and yet.

Zoo: We were the animals. They shouldn't have fed us.

Rock, Paper, Scissors
Invent Calling Shotgun

I should ride up front, says Rock,
for if another car cuts us off, the driver can
toss me at it through an open window.

I should ride up front, says Paper,
for the driver can draw a map on me
and never get lost.

No one uses paper maps anymore, says Scissors.
Ever hear of GPS? And Rock, wouldn't you
rather stay put, a little mountain?

Scissors, smashed, says, There has to be a better way to decide.
Paper, shredded into confetti, says, Decide with a shotgun.
Rock, covered by a confetti avalanche, says
                    And everyone calls me the dumb one.

Her Heart Was a Legend

In a dream I'm a young clam
and I feel a pearl on my tongue.
Like a gopher peeking through its hole,
an overweight, acned teen
spun Bessie Smith and Lead Belly
for the first time at a friend's house,
tore up her latest painting,
looked deep into those blues,

like sky like water her brown eyes bursting
to life as that music gave her a way to see.
Her sweetest, most wounded notes
broke the bars on a cage
called Port Arthur.
She glided on that river of song
hitchhiked her way onto a breeze
that blew all the way to San Francisco.

I too felt like I'd been left
at the place that raised me,
a dog abandoned who didn't belong
and sniffed its way back home
and it was "Piece of My Heart"
that shook me loose,
"Cry Baby" that made me see
my hometown and wail,

"Get It While You Can"
that made me want to get out.
Fire burns to ash and steel turns
to rust but Janis became Janus,
the coin with two faces, one peering
into darkness, listening to silence,
the other attuned only to the ragged,
dangerous song churning in her

and shadows of demons only she could see.
I have heard that earthworms have taste buds
all over their bodies and so they writhe
and twist and taste it all, and Janis
tasted it all before the worms got her,
before her demons brushed her away like barroom drunks
poking at spider webs -- $200 a day on heroin
and her Porsche speeding down Sunset Blvd.,

the winding road just another rug pulled out from under her.

Rock, Paper, Scissors Go to Therapy

In my dreams, a meteorite breaks my way, says Rock.
She sings like a statue. She laughs like a mountain.
When I wake, she goes back to the world she came from.

In my dreams, calculations cover me, says Paper.
They tell a story that ends with men
handing my green self to other men.

In my dreams, I cut paper, says Scissors,
into the shape of my mother, blades far apart,
doing a karate move called a scissor kick.

Grace

I was born a month before my country flagged
the moon. Once, young, drunk, and lonely,
I tried to follow a star but lost it in the smog.
I have seen the signs. They say, *Hell is Real,*
His and Herpes, and *Welcome to Indiana.*

The other night as dinner steamed on
our plates, I said *Dear Lord* and my son said,
Shut the Hell up once and for all and my daughter
said *Amen.* Abel God loved. Cain He hated.
Adam and Eve must have had such mixed feelings.

I keep wanting to deserve grace,
which makes no sense, I know.
Bows in her hair, smoke in her eyes,
the first girl I loved existed only in a song.
I want the other ark, the one with unicorns,

mermaids, two cyclopes gazing into each other's eye.
The pastor has writer's block because
last Sunday he overheard someone say
My favorite part of the sermon was when
it ended, and he heard someone else say *Amen.*

Dirty Looks

In my son's wide eyes I can see
the steeple of the church we left
after one too many dirty looks—
mosquito bites that you can't scratch
and soothe—when we couldn't shush him

and I can see him playing
all afternoon with a vacuum cleaner
and gazing out the window with wonder
at the gray power lines
while all the other kids
smear cake on their faces
and run through the sprinkler
at another birthday party
he didn't get invited to.

On his breath I smell mustard
that smothered his French fries tonight like
the hot dogs we bought at the ball park
when the summer sun melted him down
made him sputter *I don't need this!*
You leave me alone! as the force of his foot
made the hot bleachers shake
and people booed us,

and we whisked him and his brothers away
without asking for a refund

though we'd only hit the bottom
of the second. We couldn't face
the faces full of judgment
and pride over their kids' home runs.
*Some parents just don't know how
to discipline their kids* said some guy

to his wife. Did I flash them a smile
full of Christ-like compassion?
I didn't. I couldn't. But I also didn't
pray for God to smite them
with a hail of foul balls. I walked away,
head down like a worn-out pitcher
about to be yanked from the mound.

Skinny Dipping

My god, my body
has changed as if my old place of business
has been shuttered.
Thank you, Lord, for my body,
how it resembles a car that resembles
a coffin with wheels,
dented but not yet totaled.
My body a drowned treasure chest
picked clean by pirates. Thank you,
Gravity, for keeping me grounded,
but just once I want to be a helium balloon.
To be naked with no shame
no matter how many people point.
There's an American Association for Nude Recreation
but I'm not a joiner. I don't have a friend in the world
who would be into skinny dipping
and maybe that's what's missing.
But I won't go skinny dipping alone.
I'll be a stream that's made peace with the ocean.

I want to sing into Van Gogh's severed ear
and let him paint me nude and blue,
my face unfinished, my body a temporary address
in a town you never hear about except
when fugitive criminals get tracked down there.
I'll learn to swim in the body I have.
I promise I was young once, but too self-conscious

to dance. I should have danced, music or no music.
Now I'm the lake I dog-paddle in.
Now my body is a doorway into a room on fire.
Now my body is a framed painting my children colored over.
Sometimes I lie and dream that my body is new.
Sometimes I lie and dream of never waking.
Sometimes I write aubades that want to be gunshots.
Sometimes I think there should be more of me.
Someone in every group of skinny dippers thinks
it's funny to hide other people's clothes.
Someone always takes pictures.
The cops always arrive but never join in.

In My Man Cave

The awful silence kept going and growing
like our teenagers and our grocery bills.
My self-consciousness had fallen away like my hair.
I closed my eyes, saw a coffin open up like the lips
of the first girl I ever kissed. Mosquitos feasted on my neck
which also reminded me of the first girl I kissed,
her name gone like the title of a movie
I remember liking but don't remember.

I poured a flight of bourbons and entered the world
of a poetry anthology where I read about a sunset
that looked like a hummingbird's wings giving out
and I tasted a bourbon with hints of sour apple
and felt as forgotten as a sentence in the middle
of a technical manual, though in the background
one of our kids grunted and sweated beneath
a barbell while the others made a ping pong ball
sound like popcorn popping. More bourbon
until again I saw the first girl I ever kissed,
her body older and then gone and I said,

Hey girl, you're just a symbol of my lost youth anyway
and listened harder to the poetry
telling me my struggles, which I hold so close,
will come to a close, telling me that
before 1932, the entire world lived without
electric guitars and may have felt the lack

without really knowing what it was, just this feeling
of missing something loud and essential.
And this feeling in me, maybe it amounted to
missing something that hadn't been invented yet.

Only Son

Brother, it bothers me
to think of all the times
we got each other into trouble.
I can still hear you taking the belt
for using the good china as flying discs,
though that was my idea, born of boredom.

I can still hear you saying it wasn't you,
until Dad's enraged eyes turned to me,
and I can still feel the fear flashing through me,
and I can still hear you saying it wasn't me,
until Dad's eyes went from rage to bewilderment,

and he said both of us need to shape up,
and put his belt back on. I remember stealing
your bike and wrecking it, and I remember
borrowing your headphones so I could hear music
while you had no way not to listen to our parents

fighting it out, Mom throwing Dad out, and I remember
how you took up smoking, and how I prayed for you,
how you took up drinking, and how I worried about you,
how you got cut from the team, though I pleaded with the coach,
how you took to cutting yourself, how you stopped

eating right, stopped sleeping in the bed right
next to mine, and I ask you now to forgive me

for everything, as I forgive you now for the time
we were just single cells, swimming with all our might,
how I saw the egg and said let's go, and though you said no,

though you said no, I forgive you bro,
though I think you had the gene for shredding on guitar
and the gene for smooth-talking girls without shyness,
I understand now that you weren't ready for this world
that I've had to wander from the start as an only son.

Will Be Done

—for Will Brown

You were my student and I failed you.
And I've failed others.
Like the freshman, late for class,

music audible despite headphones,
who disrupted our reading of "do not
go gentle into that good night."

Did you rage as day broke with its peach light, Will?
Sometimes, to write, you had to go places
so dark and so silent you fell and kept falling.

On your way back to yourself,
you got lost and we lost you.
We missed you during the final, Will.

Nothing's more final than this death.
Will, this isn't really for you.
It's for everyone left.

I'm using a device called *apostrophe*.
As if you're the urn, not the ashes.
As if you're Autumn, not the fallen.

But you knew that already.
We covered it in class.
While you were still with us.

Before I smelled booze on your breath.
At two pm. Outside my office.
Before the incompletes.

Before your freshmen complained that you kept missing class.
That they missed you. I miss you.
Your life was incomplete, Will. You didn't fail.

Will you wake in another world among the stars?
Will it feel strange not having the darkness you're used to?
The darkness you used to carry everywhere?

There's light in this puddle and my face in this puddle
and when I step, there's a splash and the light goes away
and my face goes away but both return.

The light will never return to your face.
Your face will never return
to any puddle or mirror or classroom.

Everybody left came back.
You left and will not come back.
The bullet left the gun like curses from a mouth

that would eat them whole to take them back, but can't.
I'm fighting my demons, you wrote to me.
You lost your way and your battle and you broke

like one of your bottles, spirits spilling
out of every shattered, unswept piece of you.
I lost Nashville and Tennessee in my rearview mirror

and stanzas I wrote in my head but not on paper
and you, lost like Atlantis, like an old man's memories,
like a wallet, snatched on the first night in a city far from home.

I never bought that PRS Starla we checked out together
at Royal Music, and now I never will.
You said, *It's expensive*. I said, *It's overpriced*.

You said, *I could never afford it*. I said, *My wife would never allow it*.
But we both loved the bird inlays on the fretboard.
Now when I visit the music store, the birds

shriek as if impaled, kabobbed.
If I touch the guitar it will scream
every caged sound you never let out.

Every day now I listen to David Bowie sing
"Rock and Roll Suicide." *You're not alone*, he sings.
I wish I'd said that. *I've had my share*, Will.

There's a D9 chord in that song, Will.
I wish you were here to show me how to finger it.
You and your girlfriend never did come over for dinner.

Now you never will. My wife makes this teriyaki steak.
It tastes amazing. It tastes like love feels.
It tastes like the most beautiful song you ever heard.

I just reviewed *Pump Up The Volume*.
Christian Slater's underground DJ character talks on air
with a suicidal teen. The next night

he lights candles, plays "If It Be Your Will,"
by Leonard Cohen, and weeps: *I never said, "Don't do it."*
I never said that. I never said, *You're not alone.*

I'm not really talking to you, Will.
I'd just as well talk to the West Wind or an artichoke.
Everyone left, I'm talking to you. Don't leave.

You're not alone. You're not alone. You're not alone.

II. Between Worlds

The Last Time I Took
My Son to the Movies

We saw *Wonder*, the story of a boy
named Auggie with a facial deformity
caused by Treacher Collins Syndrome,
who gets bullied until the other kids
get used to his face and learn to see
past it into his beautiful true self.

My son started talking too loud.
I knew his whole script:
Our car has 162,900 miles on it.
I've saved $304. I'm buying a leaf blower,
some extension cords, some button-down shirts.
They're remodeling my high school.
They're putting in straight halls
because people get lost in the circular halls.
They should study the interactive map like I do.
How long will this movie take?

The man in front of my son turned and said, *Shut up.*
My son's face reddened. He rocked back and forth,
said, *You shut up. I'll call the police on you*
as the man tried to lock eyes with him.
I leaned forward and said, *Turn around, man.*
The man and I locked eyes with the fiercest looks
we could muster. This lasted forever, a minute, maybe.
We locked eyes for so long that my mind wandered:

Will Auggie make friends?
What is making that squeaking sound in my Toyota?
Should I take it to a mechanic?
Who was AC/DC's singer before Bon Scott?

The man pointed at my son and said, *One more time.*
I said, *Let's go right now,* and he finally turned
back to the screen, where Auggie's dad was telling him
to take off his space helmet and face this world
and the other children staring at his face.

Ten minutes later, my son was still upset,
saying, *I'll wreck you* and *You don't do that.*
The man turned again. I leaned forward again,
said, *Look, my son has special needs.*
Do you understand that we're watching a movie
about accepting people with special needs?
and my son said, *I have autism.*
The man said, *Okay. You should have said so before*
and he was right. He and his daughter found other seats.

By the end of the movie, I felt bad
for the man. He didn't know
about my son and we don't know
what he might live with: his father
newly-dead, like Malcolm Young, at age 64,
unable to remember the songs
of his own heart, his job just lost

and him wondering when he could
afford to take his daughter
to the movies again. I wanted to
take him out for a beer.
I would have listened to him
talk about his father and his daughter.
I would have tried to help him
find a job. But after the movie,
I couldn't find that man among the faces
adjusting to the lights coming on.

Adopting a Teenager
Via State Foster Care

We want a daughter, we say.
We have a girl, say the ladies with clipboards.
She's about to be hit by a bus.
She's been in many wrecks.
She's always got a break or a bruise.

She's about to be hit by a bus? we echo.
The ladies with clipboards point
at a teen girl, arms outstretched
toward an advancing bus.

We run to her. We wrap ourselves around her.
We can't stop the bus. It hits all three of us.
We wake in the hospital.
We're your parents now, we smile.

I hate you, she says.
That bus was my boyfriend.
He buys me stuffed animals.
He says he loves me and would never hurt me.
He photoshopped our faces
over a bride and groom
and he'll be sneaking in my bedroom window at night.

We've got ourselves a daughter, we say.

My Chili Recipe: An Ars Poetica

I. Whatcha Need

the river
3 pounds ground beef
the passing of the dead on the banks of what remains
4 Tbsp. minced garlic
a galloping
sound
2 diced green peppers
the sound of a violin being shattered by a perfectionist
1 diced onion
the wind, humming half-drunkenly
1 16oz. can red kidney beans
the song of nuns calming children during a hurricane
1 beer
the four seasons
1 16oz. can pinto beans
a mouth full of vowels and air
6 bay leaves
every ache in your body
2 16oz. cans of corn
thee and *thou* and *thy* and the way all three make your
tongue feel under your teeth
3 tsp. salt
Agamemnon's last cry and the sound of his spear whistling
in the Trojan wind
3 Tbsp. sugar

the long process of two people becoming a couple
1 Tbsp. chili powder
the words you need when you're untethered from yourself
3 Tbsp. Dale's seasoning sauce
the sound of that violinist trying again
2 15oz. cans diced tomatoes
the words that bring the world back when it's floating
    away like a helium balloon
1 tsp. black pepper
breaking up and making up
1 8oz. can tomato sauce
the odor of the Library of Alexandria burning
2 Tbsp. vinegar
the prayer of a dying man, veiled in anagrams
3 serrano peppers
all of your sorrows

II. Whatcha Do

Begin with the river. Brown beef and memories of the
dead with garlic, green peppers, the heartsong of the
near-shattered violinist, and onion. Love the world the
way a horse's spirit gallops in its body. Add the whistles
of wind, the nunsong, the mouthfuls of air and vowels,
the *thee* and the *thy* and the *thou*, the ache of human
pangs, the spear shivering in midair, the long process of
becoming a couple, the words you need to bring yourself
back to yourself. Add Dale's after draining grease.

Add heat and ingredients, starting with seasonings. Add the seasons. Sprinkle in sighs and songs, the sound of the violin trying again, the words you need to bring the world back to the world. Slowly bring to boil. Add beer and beans, the tide, corn, tomatoes, and tomato sauce. Add bay leaves and breakups followed by makeups. Put all of your sorrows into the anagrammed prayer and leave them there to simmer. Cook over med/low heat for two hours, stirring occasionally.

I See Your Lips Move, Lord

I don't know, Lord, but sometimes I feel
like all my accomplishments
could fit inside a Pez dispenser,
with room left over for candy.
Let my coins spilled in this world

add up to a fortune in heaven.
I've seen bricks content
to hold up other bricks. I've seen
middle managers whose bosses
called them successes, whose families

were sunshine at the soccer complex.
But you made me a brick that wished
to be a wall, and if I'd succeeded
at becoming a wall, seeing people trapped
inside or kept outside, I would have wanted

only to fall. Lord, let me fall.
Call it an accident or call it
my plan tucked inside your plan.
Verily Lord, you made me
and I made mistakes

and you filled me with ambitions
like air inspiring a balloon. *Pop*
is the sound I make calling out

to you from the torn-up dark and *crash*
is what I do in my car and my bed.

You speak. I can almost hear you.
I see your lips move
every time I see a flock
lifted by the dead distant
light of the stars.

Two-Foot Tall Poem

I'm in a homey coffee shop in a strange town
next door to a famous indie bookstore
that's supposed to be open but isn't,
and I'm shopping for images, as Ginsberg would have it,
searching for inspiration, as it were,
when this toddler toddles up to my table
and says, *Hi*, over and over, like fifty times,
or maybe he's saying, *high*, because honestly
he's behaving like a meth head who just got
out of a mental hospital, but it's okay because he's little,

so I smile at his mom and sit still in an effort to convey
that I'm a friendly stranger, patient, kid-loving,
but not a creepy stranger, candy in pockets, kid-loving
in a whole other, disturbing way, but I'm thinking
maybe she should pull him away, teach him wariness,
and I'm thinking he's interrupting my creative process,
as it were, but then I remember another coffeeshop
where I saw a minister of my acquaintance
at a table with some college students,
when a meth head just out of a mental hospital

approached their table, and the minister, who always
seemed creepy to me, who, as it turns out,
was actually committing adultery with an intern,
one of the folks at that very table, said, to the meth
    head/mental patient,
We're praying here, even though their eyes were all open,

and you've got me, I invented the meth head/mental patient
it was me approaching their table, just to say, *hi*, but also
because I was going through some shit, I forget what, exactly,
one way or another going through life like a bug
that had just been stepped on and was trying to avoid

getting stepped on again and smushed entirely,
and I remember thinking I could be the answer to their prayer
if the prayer was *Dear Lord, bring us someone in need
of being ministered to*, as I did feel the need for some
ministration, and thinking of that coffeeshop
while sitting in this coffeeshop, I realize that this kid
is my poem, a two-foot tall poem, hitting its head
on my table, then crawling back to his mom,
who now scowls at me like I'm some god
who could have kept her son, or my own, safe.

What Will Survive

Sunlight wrapped around a violet like a bejeweled dress.

Shards of ice float on a river, mirrors for clouds to shave by.

Every atom belonging to me, to you, but not our yen for dollars.

Scorpions, who can slow their metabolism to survive on
    one insect per year.

Music, that holy silence just after ceasefire.
        Gloria Gaynor's "I Will Survive"
                but not the band Survivor.

Social class distinctions, but not social distancing.

Shaky hands finally settling down. But the handshake?

Ants, who kill the infected before a virus can spread
    across their hill.

Mountains and their coldness, their hardness, their way of
    shaping breath into prayer.

The human heart, unharmed, though homeless as a hermit crab.

Keith Richards.

The echo of church bells.

The television show "Survivor" but not television.

Questions will survive. But what about declarations?

Smooth stones sung to by rain.

Raindrops sunbathing on smooth stones.

Twinkies, but probably not our custom of eating
    birthday cake after someone blows out candles.

The cadences of cockroaches and mud minnows.
        Also Larkin's line *What will survive of us is love*
          tattooed on whatever skin is left to find.

Rock, Paper, Scissors Reminisce

My best day, said Rock, was the day a child
said, "What a good rock," and picked me up,
and held me, and hurled me across the playground.

My best day, said Paper, was the day a bride
and groom printed their wedding program on me,
and held me, and took their picture with me.

My best day, said Scissors, was the day they
sharpened my blades on a rock and handed me
to a child, to cut paper. I can still hear the ripriprip.

Stars in My Beard

Wade out into night
catch you some stars,
the music said to me
as the singer/guitarist at the bar
shook out the last lonely arpeggios
and my wife at home dreamed she could lift
a fallen log off of our kids
at the same moment
as this new song made me think of her
waist-long hair when we were young
at another long-ago rock show.
Call it noise. Call it one sure way
to feel alive. The singer's red high heel
dangled above the edge of the small stage
then dropped, apple, wind-picked
last year's worries flung
into the mosh pit to be trampled
and she stayed on stage
guitar humming that this would be the year
she prevised in the pawn shops of Duluth,
fumbling for notes on a guitar
to match the ones in her head.
Her song made a space for itself
in the night, floated,
joyously there but soon gone,
smooth stone a child skips
across a pond.

Love Me Gentlefirm the Way
Firemen Love a Treed Cat

Love me when I'm world weary, when I feel like
anyone who loves me must be wrong,
when I tell you that you're mistaken, that I'm a mistake.
Love me when I feel like I'm simultaneously a door with
   no handle
and the frightened thing that can't find its way out.

Love me with your hands like I'm all the money
you can grab, with your mouth like it's happy hour—
drinks half off—with your whole body which feels
like a river when I feel like a fish, several hooks in me
like prized scars. Love me by kissing my scars.

Love me on your hands and knees like a tatterdemalion
on a desert island scooping up a bottle with a message in it.
Let your love for me be uncharted, unchartable, off the charts.
Love me blind as justice. Love me blinder than a gigantic
   roosting bat,
satisfied with a thousand mosquitos in its stomach.

Love me in golden afternoon light, in the darkness
behind your eyelids behind your sleep mask.
Love me in every room in our house, in every note
of every song you write. Love me like I'm a bookmark
holding your favorite page in your favorite book.

Love me when I spill beer on the book I borrowed
from you and sheepishly return it. Love me until your love
for me makes the ceiling spin, makes you sweat cold,
makes you need to lie down, makes your head pound, until
you swear you'll never love me this much ever again but
then you do.

My Sadness Swallows Up My Dreams

The porcupine can't help its prickly quills.
Don't blame me. Blame the shooter, says the gun.
The stars did not ask to be dead, or still,
or far away. I'm who I am, my love.

Your name's a country song stuck in my throat.
Or I'm a shadow that must follow you.
Maybe I'm spam, a scam, a junk mail note.
Or do you want to read me? Say, *I do.*

My sadness swallows up my dreams. I swim
in seas of sadness, where you are the land.
In time I reach you, beaten, tired. In
the time it takes my eyes to blink, I spend

what feels like years beside you, months, or weeks,
your long hair in my mouth, sun on your cheeks.

Fifty

All morning I gather the parts of me.
A wedding ring lodges beneath a swollen knuckle.
At least I'm not in one of those old bodies
that chases young bodies, a bird that doesn't recognize
the window between himself and that sweet parakeet.
On the other hand, my other hand writes
and remembers how to grip a tennis racquet.
My feet search for socks to cram themselves into
like songs into three radio-friendly minutes.
My mouth is an open door, my throat a foyer,
my belly a rec room. Bring more chairs, more chairs.
Earlier, my ear tried to alert me
to a new way to disappear, but it was fooling itself—
I'm a noise that's not going anywhere.
At least my eyes have stayed in my head,
which, at least, has held onto some hair.
Once a year I give blood like a Christmas present
I hope to get back. Aches ride up and down
the elevator of my body, unsure what floor
to settle on. Read the label. Side effects
may include loss of speed, memory, and parents.
My students ogle their phones rather than watch
me come apart like a cloud of smoke.
I tell them to savor each breath the way
an alcoholic savors the last shot in the bottle.
Class, one minute you're playing egg toss;
the next minute you're the egg.

At the Intersection of Yawn and Yawp

An octopus has three hearts and nine brains
is the kind of thought that enters my mind
when I'm trying to sleep, when falling asleep
seems like a magic trick, and when I try
to count sheep, the sheep turn to words
wandering in all directions as my brain and body
have awkward conversations about difficult
or pointless topics and I worry that if I succeed
at falling asleep I will doze through
my one shot at heroism or immortality
like there's a child nearby poised to be pushed
out of the way of an onrushing car
or maybe the lyrics of my one great song
have chosen this evening to hit me
like lightning but instead of gathering them
I'll have dreams that I won't remember,
and of course these worries keep me
from falling asleep, though they don't quite
keep me awake, just idling at the intersection
of yawn and yawp, a wild creature fighting
a mild teacher for the wheel, which locks up,
along with the brakes, and in the headlights a child
who turns out to be me, too, so I guess I've fallen
asleep after all, fallen for that old trick
of the imagination which says I can be the hero
as well as the child as well as the one steering,
each of my three hearts filled with magic.

Between Worlds

"I listen: sky and daisies burlesque each other,
bivouacked between worlds."
　　　　　—James Tate *"In My Own Backyard"*

On the middle of a bridge, I forget
where I was going, where I came from.

The bridge is burning
beautifully
on both ends.

The cloudless sky calls to me
through the voice of a bird,
its beak open wide as the body
of a fish being gutted.

The water below looks so coolly refreshing.

A fish leaps, plunks.

The water rushes to cover this up
like a secret.

The splash reaches the tip of my tongue.

It is a name I can't quite remember.

I forget whether I belong
to the river　　or to the sky.

Ankylosing Spondylitis

"What's Your Pain Level on a Scale of 1-10?"

1. This week six different medical paraprofessionals and three computers asked me for my date of birth. My date of birth hurts because it will be forgotten, and the date of my death hurts.

2. My hips feel like an accordion that a demon monkey is playing.

3. My back feels like an egg with a baby pterodactyl inside trying to claw its way out. I mean *I couldn't be better.*

4. MRI, DMV, and department meeting all on the same day as my manuscript gets rejected.

5. When *Everybody Hurts* by REM comes on the radio, I want to punch Michael Stipe in the nuts and force him, at gunpoint, to sing the chorus again. I feel like what that chorus would sound like.

6. Like a version of *Ground Hog Day* in which Bill Murray's character was in a car accident yesterday but has to go to work today anyway. I mean *I'm fine, and you?*

7. Sort of the physical equivalent of the distress I felt when some dude filmed and distributed nudes of my daughter.

8. You don't want to know. I mean *I'm good, thanks.*

9. I feel the way that dude who sold nudes of my daughter would have felt if I'd caught up with him, knowing I could exact revenge with no legal penalties.

10. You really don't want to know.

If This Next Apocalypse
Gets Canceled or Postponed

Oh Dear, can we busy ourselves trying to guess the words
    in a postcard sent by a pilot to himself at his next destination?

Can we patent a method of trading places with our
    reflections in the mirror?

I want to prove that San Antonio is the receptionist's desk
    at a summer resort for angels.

Let's go to an unfamiliar city at night, and let's get so hungry
    and tired that the squeaking room service cart
        makes a music more beautiful than Brahms.

Let's let the different words for yearning die on our tongues
    as if they've just stung the different words for satisfied.

Can we find words for every feeling that our cleverness can't
    comprehend, every thought we can't express when awake?

Can we live like somewhere in the future we sit, dazed and amazed,
    remembering what we did today, wishing we could reach
        into the past to give ourselves a high five?

Let's plot a way to die with the dignity of a snowman
    and the raccoon frozen inside its torso.

Let's sleep with the window open, with the scent of lavender,
   with the sound of rain stunning our restored hearts.

I want to prove that gray skies and rain were born
      when God finally did the dishes and drained the sink
         after a hard night of making and unmaking.

Let's climb into this wreckage and let the night be
      a story that keeps dreaming itself,
            a new beginning, a better middle, and in the end,

your name running just past my ability to say it.

III. A World Inside This World

A World Inside This World

I love watching Bigfoot
in the famous Patterson film,
glance cast over her shoulder
as if at a sudden takeoff of birds,
arms swinging in time to some mysterious
rainforest music, no need to break
stride before returning to her
own thoughts and the ground before her.
So what if all the evidence shows
she is just a man in a suit?

All the evidence shows that I too
am just a man in a suit,
too hurried to walk like that
or even like the young – unsteady, unsure
where they're going but with years
to get there. My size ten Rockports
already look small next to the size eleven
Converses my fourteen-year-old autistic son
got for Christmas. His enthusiasm for fashion
is legendary, as is his passion for the smallest,
most surprising things. Every day he tells me
how many button-down shirts
he owns (twenty-three at last count).
Every day he says, *Guess what,*
I've been in high school for 91 days,
92 days, 93 days, 94 days, Wow!

Dickinson wrote, *The heart has many doors,*
and on the rare occasion when my son lets me in
his room to show me, once again, a You Tube video
of the ten fastest race cars, or to tell me snakes
move twelve miles per hour, I feel I've entered
a secret, mythical place, where my son rules everything
in shouting distance, and it's okay to shout in his world,
okay to repeat a name a hundred times
because the syllables taste so sweet,
okay to bay and rage without pretension
or say just what's on your mind even if it's been there
for months and you've been saying it over and over,
and typical ways of seeing the world
seem like cubic zirconia dreams I've been sold
that keep me from smelling
what Wallace Stevens called the *odor of stars,*
from finding a world inside this world.

Then my son says, *That's enough.*
He needs to walk alone. My presence
threatens to despoil his forest.
I walk out, once again exiled from my own heart,
GPS signal lost, contacts gone,
habitual ways of seeing the world
knocked to the floor like books from a coffee table.
I never would have believed before this
that such a creature could ever exist.

If You've Met One Autistic Person, You've Met One Autistic Person

—popular saying within the ASD support community

My son's the only person that I know
who thinks this way, who acts this way.
The boy eats three potatoes every day.
He says he wants to gain weight, wants to grow

his waist. To keep from melting down, he'll throw
ice cubes across our yard. A game. Who plays?
My son's the only person. That I know.
Who thinks this way? Who acts this way?

Who asks how much you weigh? How fast you'll grow?
Who says whatever their heart says to say?
Don't let him bend to suit the world, I pray.
Who dreams up paths where no one else can go?
My son's the only person that I know.

An Urn Among Music Boxes

I.
My dad is made of balsa wood.
He's wider than he is tall,
taller than he is deep.

On his face, you can read
"Footprints," the sentimental poem
that everyone's mom sticks on the fridge.

My dad has Non-Hodgkins Lymphoma.
Roundup® from the farm next door infected him.
First an allergic reaction to meds
made his tongue swell up, gave him a rash.
Then came tests. Then came the diagnosis.

In the hospital, he couldn't talk
except by spelling on a board.
A machine breathed for him.
He ate through a tube in his nose.

If you open him up and turn the key,
inoffensive music should come out.
It's my task to open him up, turn the key,

and listen, knowing the music will wind down.

II.

I guess I retire from Walmart,
my dad wrote from his hospital bed,
but nothing could make him quit

flea markets, so here we are,
my sisters and I, lifting boxes,
arranging inventory on tables

like kids again doing whatever Dad says—
hard work but also a cakewalk
started and stopped by the rhythmic

orders coming from Dad's still-damaged voice.

III.

Last night, in the deep fog on 234E,
two deer galloped in front of my car
and I had to swerve to miss them

as Lou Reed music set my stereo reeling.

IV.

Test each music box, my dad says.
If there's no music, don't put it on the table.
If the glass is broken, don't put it on the table.

Dad, this one's not a music box.
It's an urn. It has instructions
on the bottom for storing ashes

and no music comes out.
My dad says, *Morticians charge*
for those. $5 per music box.

$10 for the urn. My dad's a music box.
My sisters and I are music boxes, too.
We're also hard workers, and this is a cake walk,

and when the music stops, someone will land in the urn.

   V.
At 8am, a vendor, crossing the street
to get something from her car
gets hit by a vehicle going 50 mph.

I hear it and hope it isn't my car
getting hit. Then I hear *Ohmigod*
and *Get up, Mama*, and minutes later

a lady holding a coffee maker
asks, *Will you take $3?*
and my dad takes her money as

his friend Shawn directs traffic,
and an ambulance comes,
as does a helicopter like the one

that airlifted my dad two months ago
and a teenage girl, trying to figure out
which music box to have her boyfriend

buy for her, opens several boxes
at once, and there's this cacophony
of chimes, and my dad says,

Quit standing around, son. We've got work to do.

Don't Try

—inscription on Charles Bukowski's tombstone

I wanted to be a drummer who wanted
to be a drum but I always felt more
like the broken string that ruined the song
and scared off the Sub Pop execs.
Wound up tight until I snapped.
Nostalgia, you dirty window.
Look, my first grunge show, Seattle 1991,
head hairy, arms skinny, taking a dive
from the stage at The Off Ramp
deciding then and there not to try
any more lest I be called *poser*.

At University of Washington I wrote
essays, but I found that too trying.
Also tiring. My kids have never
heard the word *poser* but if one studies
too much the others call him a *try-hard*.
It would be a bummer to become a bum
and I wish I could go back and slam dance
at the Moore Theater to live Nirvana
but first I'd shout into the mic that 2021 smells
like Teen Spirit mixed with the un-washable
funk of middle age and sounds like the moment

after the encore and before the applause. Time
is a wind that will pick your pocket, especially if

you're a screaming tree in a garden of sound.
The world now is a peaceful battlefield
after the casualties on one side rise
from their bodies and help up the casualties
on the other side like sweaty moshers
clad in black concert tees lifting
fallen fellow moshers in the pit.
None can remember why they started
shooting and they'd hug if they still had bodies.

To Make Light of the Dark

For now I can live face down,
pants unbuttoned, ass exposed,
nurses and doctors scurrying about,
discussing the song on the radio,
how it reminds them of a tv show
now off the air, and I guess I can
even live through "Rate your pain
on a scale of 1-10" and
"What's your date of birth?"

As the needle plunges into my hip,
I can live knowing my wings
are vestigial and no one believes
I can hear them flap when I lie like this
on a table or when I lie like this: *I feel fine.*

And I can live knowing I'll leave
this world I've stumbled through,
often lost in something or someone.
I'll leave like sherbet melting.
I'll leave like a match fizzling out.
But I can't bear the thought that the words
I've found to make light of the dark
won't leave a mark more lasting
than a dent on a dead man's pillow.

Body Breaking

Walking is a mound of clothes that don't fit any more,
running, a page scrawled all over, crumpled.

Though my diseased body feels as unlovable
as a family of rats,

will she still cherish me the way a musician
cherishes a vintage instrument?

Who am I, legs no longer carrying me to places
closed to me now like raging fists?

Icarus half-drowned, head still in the clouds, but balding,
sunburned, scratched half-raw.

The Man I Hoped to Be

The man I hoped to be just killed himself.
The man I hoped to be just killed himself.
The words I tried to write have self-erased.
The words I tried to write have self-erased.
The man has self-erased. The words killed him.
I tried to hope. I just write to be.

A student says I don't know how to teach.
A student says I don't know how to teach.
Our wayward daughter's on the road again.
Our wayward daughter's on the road again.
I don't know how to teach our wayward daughter.
A student says *On the Road* again?

I'm only grounded when I'm in your arms.
I'm only grounded when I'm in your arms.
My way to fly's to hide in your long hair.
My way to fly's to hide in your long hair.
I'm only in your arms to hide. In your long hair
I'm grounded when my way's to fly.

Just say your student's killed himself a fly.
I tried to write the man I hoped to be.
Our wayward daughter's grounds have self-erased.
I'm armed when on my way to teach.
Again, I don't know how to hide.
I'm in the only road, in your long hair.

Upon First Reading *Jesus'*
Son by Denis Johnson

The linings of my veins
ached in the middle
of a warfare of noises.
What was going to happen
rained down on my head.
I hadn't wanted to find the man
hanging what he was dreaming
so that the air pulsed with color.
I was going home from
some basic misunderstanding.
Like a foreigner breathing,
seeds were moaning in the gardens.

I was so flooded with yearning
a spasm ran through me.
Light streaks striped Tom's face.
I was out of luck, a china cup
in millions of bits, but happy
like a machine that polishes stones.
The sky didn't have any shadows in it.

And the Savior did come, but
right now he is, I think, in the state
prison in Colorado. Like the dead
coming back, a mist covered everything.
I felt the beauty, a deep thirst being quenched.

That world! These days it's all brainless
angels bruised the colors of a tattoo.
Sunset danced on my despair.
The torn moon mended.

I was in love, enough to drink
for two hours. I staggered, clinging
to a book. Most days are crushed
breathless by something far away,
too beautiful, true in a fiery
and glorious way. I was born
in a story, word for word,
alive in a deeper sense,
coming back over and over.
Look in the mirror. Hah!
Wrecked cars. My bullet hole.

Nothing could stifle the blurry music
of rush hour absorbing the sounds of my steps
full of smoke and silences I didn't want to hear.
My guts jumping with unintelligible words,
I heard lovely cries, music, messages.
I heard the world smolder
around its edges for a heartbeat.

There might be a place for people like us.

Rock, Paper, Scissors Want to be Called . . .

Call me Gem,
says Rock,
smoother than
a skipping stone,
harder than
black coal.

Call me Parchment,
says Paper.
It's like calling
a person
Doctor
or Boss.

Call me like a bell calling your kids to dinner,
says Scissors. See, I have two legs, and I'm small.
Call me Ish. Call me Mael. Don't call me
late. Don't call me for dinner.
Call me like a suicide hotline
when you feel alone, when you think about cutting.

It's Not So Hard to Write a Sonnet, Man

It's not so hard to write a sonnet, Man.
Write of a loving couple paired like rhyme.
Let them get old, but not their love, and scan
your lines so that they dance in time,

the lines, I mean, but yes, the lovers, too.
And let them fight. Let them go broke and break
each other down in ways you never knew
that lines and hearts could break. Let each one take

a turn at burning down what they have made
together. Let them make/remake their love.
You may need to revise. Don't be afraid
of amniotic fluid, tears, or blood.

A sonnet's not so hard to write, my friend.
What's hard is loving so love doesn't end.

I Regret Caring More About What People Think Than About People

At the high school reunion, I intended
  to confess an old crush—cliché, I know—
and there she was, lovely as I remembered,

  except for a blue sadness in her eyes.
Had it always been there? The gilded
  picture frame around her face, the candle

burning in front of the picture frame,
  and the obituary, also framed, told me she'd
OD'd along with Mr. Most Likely to Succeed.

  I regretted being too chicken to risk
her breaking my heart, him breaking my face.
  Her beauty and his muscles had been

a "members only" sign and a cross-armed
  bouncer at a club I convinced myself
I could never enter. I regretted not taking her

  in my teenage twig arms
and telling her that together we could invent
  happiness

and share it with our classmates
  who couldn't even fake it well
at the balding, sagging reunion.

I regretted the hours lost
to a computer screen, the questions
    I didn't ask about the faces

staring back at me, the online arguments
    with people who would have clicked "like"
if I'd said *Help, there's a sunset outside*

    and I should be flying through
the rush and ache of it but I'm stuck
    slow-dying in this terminal.

I would like to jail the part of me
    that trained the wild dogs in my heart
to sit, to lie down, to stay.

    I regret those high school dances
where I lurked in the darkness, afraid
    of my own dance moves, hidden

as a tree in a forest, swaying
    no more nor less than the rest,
not yet aware that its branches hold birds

    made of beautiful songs that could
rise just before a wildfire
    torches everything in sight.

Downloadable Caffeine

—For David Berman, 1967-2019

*"All this new technology / will eventually give us new
feelings / that will never completely displace the old
ones, / leaving everyone feeling quite nervous / and
split in two."*
                              —David Berman, "Self-Portrait at 28"

Let's celebrate the coffee hour, when the day
could still take a right turn or a left turn or turn out
better than okay or at least better than yesterday.
Sunlight might splash on your face and you
might hear Nashville in a stone skipping
or in the voices of those whose blood runneth orange.

Let's call these Winning Lottery Tickets before
we scratch them, in the coffee hour, Realm of Could-Be,
because singing a song into existence feels like
injecting a new narcotic called Bridge-Between-Us
because I have been listening to David Berman for years
and strumming a guitar that wouldn't let me learn to play it.

Let's say a garage band opens the door for air
as they work on Silver Jews covers: "Pretty Eyes,"
"Send in the Clouds," and "I Remember Me."
Let's say it's a real garage door and not a metaphor.
Metaphors are a radical invention. They connect us.
Metaphors are O.G. cell phones. Welcome, world of

thousands of friends with whom I'll never shake hands
or share a hug. Welcome, awkward feelings that won't leave,
because the present feels like 66% past and 33% future,
and if you wake thinking *knowing anything with certainty*
feels like lifting an automobile off a wounded poodle
and a phrase from a tabloid headline rolls around your head,

let me tell you again about the night I saw a cover band
play a Silver Jews set at The End in Nashville,
how Bob Nastanovich and David Berman showed up,
Bob all goofy charm, David humble and nervous and split.
I wish I could go back, plug that music and that night
into myself, inject a heavy dose of song or let it fill my cup.

"and pain will be the thing that saves us."

> *"When Illness Is Cure"*
> —Bob Hicok

I had to write a sex scene for my screenplay, and
I had her say "oh baby!" as he, in a cry of sweet pain
said "yes, baby!" but I know what he doesn't, that she will
get pregnant tonight, and I know this baby will be
different than planned, someday a Special Olympian, not the
pro prospect they've hoped for. Often the thing
you say is the same thing someone else says even as that
thing means something different, the way *saves*
can be a baseball term, can precede *money*, can follow *Jesus*.

Rock, Paper, Scissors
Celebrate the End of the War

A wind ran right over me and climbed through a window,
says Rock. No more windows for me. I'm retired.
In peacetime, I can be some poet's pet.

They erased their battle plans off me, says Paper,
and wrote a treaty on that clean slate. Fold me
into an airplane. I feel so zig-zaggingly free.

From now on, I will cut only ribbons,
says Scissors. The war, unlike me,
never had a point.

Questions for Further Study

How are these poems like dark dad jokes with Gillette®
razors in them and wild slept-on hair and a receding
hairline, all the punchlines lost like a wedding ring
swallowed by a toddler sitting on a potty chair learning that
this is going to hurt us more than it hurts you is just one of life's
pretty lies, like the one about birdsong and poetry both
being peaceful and chime-like, when really both are
elaborate ways of saying *let's get it on* or *stay out of my tree*?

Is it possible to write something original about turning fifty?
What would Keats have written about turning fifty had he
turned fifty? Will my name be written on ice with spray
paint or carved into a tree next to my wife's name or
whispered into our grandkids' ears soft as snow falling on
the wings of a dead bird?

What is the symbolism of the light in the puddle, the
Buffalo-shaped ache? The soap bubble? The skipping stone?
If the author were truly a good father, would he for real
compare his kids to Bigfoot or write similes like flashlights
shining in their eyes?

Have you or anyone you know made it through
Remembrances of Things Past? Have you felt the loss of
someone you never really knew? Have you seen through the
color blue into its constituents, magenta and cyan? Have
you felt like there's something wrong with you but you
never knew what until you read about it in a book and if so

did you hate the book and its author or did you feel
grateful like the time you were about to sing "The Star
Spangled Banner" before a baseball game with toilet
paper clinging to your shoe when a bat boy jogged up to
you, pointed out the toilet paper, pulled it off, and
disposed of it in the dugout?

Do these words move across your heart a) like
tumbleweeds across a desert b) like wind gusts blown in
from the sea or c) like the beautiful new person at work
who gets promoted before learning your name?
Where children are concerned is it fair to say that the
heart is Santa's sleigh weighed down by an impossible
load, the heart a small thing dragged across the night by
     large animals?

Is adopting a scared teenager more like trying to garden
on a scarred battlefield or like insisting on the day-olds at
Dunkin' Donuts? Is it like rescuing meat from a grinder in
some kind of PETA-inspired intervention and then trying
with all you have not to become the meat, not to become
     the grinder?

Is autism the beginning of a new stage of consciousness?
What would you say to the loneliest whale in the world if
he could hear or understand you if you could hear his
lonely 52-Hertz cry just lower than the lowest note on a
tuba inaudible even to other whales?

Is it possible to die from a broken heart? To dream yourself into a better self? To have an allergic reaction to water? What is the probability of being born? One in 400 trillion according to some guy on the Internet. Wow! Here we are somehow IRL and on the WWW. How does anyone ever yawn, and why can't we all live every moment in awe like Adam at the moment when he first saw Eve or like the first Cro-Magnon to gaze at a bison and paint it on the cave wall?

Acknowledgments

Versions of some of these poems were previously published in literary journals. Thanks to the editors of those journals.

The American Journal of Poetry: "Will Be Done"

Another Chicago Magazine (ACM): "If This Next Apocalypse Gets Canceled or Postponed," "Love as the World Ends"

B O D Y: "Two-Foot Tall Poem," "Ankylosing Spondylitis"

Book of Matches: "And Pain Will Be the Thing That Saves Us"

The Chaffin Journal: "I Never Pushed My Daughter," "Stars in My Beard"

Chiron Review: "Adopting a Teenager Via State Foster Care"

Concho River Review: "I Regret Caring More About What People Think Than About People"

Crazyhorse: "The Last Time I Took My Son to the Movies"

Eastern Iowa Review: "Love Me Gentlefirm the Way Firemen Love a Treed Cat"

Kentucky Philological Review: "Upon First Reading *Jesus' Son* by Denis Johnson"

Literary Accents: "My Chili Recipe (An *Ars Poetica*)"

Louisville Review: "Fifty"

The MacGuffin: "The Man I Hoped to Be"

Michigan Quarterly Review: "Dear God, Show Me How to Walk in Wonder"

The Midwest Quarterly: "Her Heart Was a Legend," "Rock, Paper, Scissors Reminisce"

Miracle Monocle: "Downloadable Caffeine"

North Dakota Review: "A World Inside This World"

One Art: "An Urn among Music Boxes," "Don't Try," "Skinny Dipping"

Parabola: "Grace"

The Penn Review: "In My Man Cave"

Pine Hills Review: "What Will Survive"

Rattle: "If You've Met One Autistic Person, You've Met One Autistic Person," "People Yawn When Other People Yawn"

Reformed Journal: "I See Your Lips Move, Lord"

San Antonio Review: "Dirty Looks"

SmokeLong Quarterly: "Questions for Further Study"

Valparaiso Poetry Review: "It's Not so Hard to Write a Sonnet, Man"

Waxwing: "Remember Those Girls, Lord"

Yearling Poetry Journal: "Only Son"

"If You've Met One Autistic Person, You've Met One Autistic Person" was reprinted in *Imaginative Writing: The Elements of Craft*, ed. Janet Burroway (Pearson Education, 2024).

"It's Not So Hard to Write a Sonnet, Man" was reprinted in *How to Write a Form Poem,* ed. Tania Runyan (T.S. Poetry Press, 2020).

"My Chili Recipe (An *Ars Poetica*)" and "Questions for Further Study" were reprinted in *Fantastic Imaginary Creatures,* ed. Gerry LaFemina (Madville Publishing, 2023).

"Will be Done" was reprinted in *The Poetry Gymnasium: 110 Proven Exercises to Shape Your Best Verse,* ed. Tom C. Hunley (McFarland, 2019).

"Dear God, Show Me How to Walk in Wonder" was featured on *Verse Daily* on June 18, 2023.

"Fifty" was featured on *Verse Daily* on May 7, 2021.

"If You've Met One Autistic Person, You've Met One Autistic Person" was featured on *Verse Daily* on December 7, 2021.

"People Yawn When Other People Yawn" was featured on *Verse Daily* on 7/28/2020.

"The Last Time I Took My Son to the Movies" was reprinted in *Verse Daily* on Janurary 25, 2021.

Versions of the following poems were published in *Adjusting to the Lights*, winner of the 2020 *Rattle* Chapbook Prize: "Dear God, Show Me How to Walk in Wonder," "Dirty Looks," "I Never Pushed My Daughter," "The Last Time I Took My Son to the Movies" "Remember Those Girls, Lord," and "A World Inside This World."

"Questions for Further Study" won the $200 *SmokeLong Quarterly* Microfiction Award at AWP 2020.

Thanks to early readers: Curtis L. Crisler, Rachel Custer, the lovely Ralaina Hunley, Greg Kosmicki, Luke Johnson, Lee Rossi, Bianca Stone, Mathias Svalina, and Amy Wright.

About the Author

Tom C. Hunley is the author of *Adjusting to the Lights* (Rattle Chapbook Prize, 2020), *What Feels Like Love: New and Selected Poems* (C&R Press, 2021), and the short film *You're Not Alone*, from Forerunner TV. He has published in such literary journals as *Atlanta Review, Crazyhorse, TriQuarterly,* and *Zone 3*. His work has also been featured on *Verse Daily, The Writer's Almanac, Poetry Daily,* and Billy Collins' *The Poetry Broadcast*. He is a professor of English and Creative Writing at Western Kentucky University, where he has taught since 2003.

www.tomchunley.com

Printed in the USA
CPSIA information can be obtained
at www.ICGtesting.com
CBHW020432060224
4090CB00005B/26